Natural Home Remedies

For Common Health Problems

RON KNESS

ISBN-13: 978-1981366019
ISBN-10: 1981366016

Contents

Disclaimer

We hope you enjoy reading our report, however we do suggest you read our disclaimer. All the material written in this document is provided for informational purposes only and is general in nature.

Every person is a unique individual and what has worked for some or even many may not work for you. Any information perceived as advice by must be considered in light of your own particular set of circumstances.

The author or person sharing this information does not assume any responsibility for the accuracy or outcome of your use of the content.

Every attempt has been made to provide well researched and up to date content at the time of writing. Now all the legalities have been taken care of, please enjoy the content.

See your healthcare professional before starting any diet, health or exercise program!

Introduction

There are many illnesses and ailments that tend to be thought of, and even diagnosed, as "conditions" rather than diseases. This is because in themselves, they are not considered to be fatal or even dangerous.

Some of them, however, may be indicators of something more serious. Some may increase in severity if left untreated, or even allow more dangerous secondary conditions to develop.

Those considerations aside, at best many of these "conditions" or "health problems" can, at the very least, cause pain, discomfort, distress and embarrassment. They make life harder and less enjoyable than it otherwise could be.

Many people are reluctant to seek treatment for these conditions, either because of their personal nature or because they don't consider them serious enough, so they put up with the symptoms, which may be continual, or may be recurring or spasmodic.

This book discusses ten health problems that overall affect a great many people. For each one there is a very brief overview of the condition and its causes, with most of the focus on easily procured and prepared natural treatments that you can do at home that have proven effective for other sufferers.

Natural Remedies for Excessive Sweating (Hyperhidrosis)

Sweating is nature's way of regulating your body temperature. Hyperhidrosis is a condition that causes sweating excessively beyond what is required to regulate body temperature. The condition may cause avoidance of certain activities or socializing due to the embarrassment or anxiety it may cause.

Excess sweating may occur over the entire body or in just certain areas such as the underarms, face, soles of the feet and palms of the hands. If your episodes of hyperhidrosis only affect your feet and hands, you may typically have only one occurrence per week, and during the hours that you're awake.

Primary and Secondary Hyperhidrosis

Primary hyperhidrosis is a type of excess sweating that has no particular medical cause. In this type of excess sweating, your sweat glands are triggered by the nerves and is likely hereditary.

Secondary hyperhidrosis is caused by a medical or health condition. The possible causes are many but include diabetes, anxiety disorder, heat exhaustion, overactive thyroid glands and menopause.

Fortunately, there are some readily available natural remedies that can produce great results, helping to control hyperhidrosis and improve your quality of life.

Some Natural Hyperhidrosis Remedies

Lemon – Apply lemon to the affected areas before you go to bed at night.

Apple Cider Vinegar – Mix with a small amount of water and apply to affected areas.

Witch Hazel – This is another great remedy. Simply apply to the affected areas.

Black Tea – This type of tea contains tannic acid that can help reduce sweating. Simply place a tea bag in warm water to soak for a few minutes and then use the tea on your hands and feet – or use the teabags for your underarms.

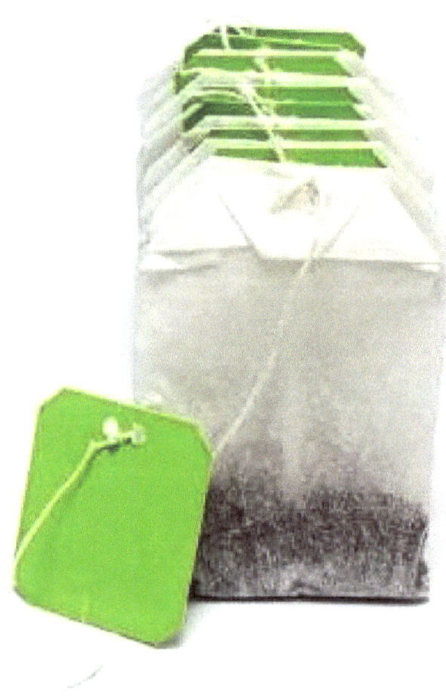

Coconut Oil – A popular remedy for many conditions of the skin, coconut oil is also very effective in reducing excess sweating. Rub the coconut oil on the affected areas of the body until it is absorbed by your skin.

Wheatgrass – Contains nutrients that help to neutralize the body's pH and prevent excess sweating. Among the many nutrients found in wheatgrass are Vitamin C, Folic Acid, protein, Vitamin B6 and Vitamin B12.

Tomato Juice – A very effective method to help hyperhidrosis because of the many healthy properties it contains. You can either purchase prepared tomato juice or prepare it yourself to make a more natural drink. Drink a glass every day.

Water – Nothing can replace water when it comes to hydrating your body and overcoming excess sweating. Water gets rid of toxins in your body and even helps reduce anxiety and stress issues which can cause hyperhidrosis.

Potato – The potato is a great remedy for excess sweating. It naturally balances your pH levels to reduce the amount of sweat produced by the glands. Clean the potato and cut into slices, then rub the slices on the affected areas.

Some medications may cause excessive sweating. Blood pressure medications, antibiotics, supplements, dry mouth medications and some psychiatric drugs may trigger or exacerbate your bouts of hyperhidrosis.

While sweating is desired during an intensive workout -- it can be embarrassing if you're in a meeting or on a date. There are many natural routes you can take to get reduce both the incidence and degree of hyperhidrosis, so keep trying if you don't succeed the first time.

Natural Remedies for Gout

Gout is a very painful form of arthritis, resulting from an excess of uric acid build-up in the body. This occurs when the kidneys are overloaded and have a hard time trying to eliminate the excess. As a result, these uric acid deposits can become crystallized and accumulate in between the joints.

Those afflicted with gout are often found to have uric acid deposits in their big toe joints. These uric acid deposits may appear as lumpy patches under the skin, and the build-up may also develop into kidney stones.

Gout can be so debilitating that even a bed sheet draped over the toe can cause excruciating pain.

Dietary changes, including reduced alcohol intake, will reduce the incidence of gout attacks. Appropriate lifestyle changes can prevent a re-occurrence. However, for those either not able or prepared to make changes, remedial treatments are available. Natural treatment options have given many relief from gout pain, here are a few.

Cherries

Cherries is one of the classic natural gout remedies. There are some gout sufferers who say it works and others say it doesn't help them. Research reveals that those who do consume cherries were found to have lowered levels of uric acid as well as a reduction in inflammation.

Either way, they are delicious and worth a try! You'll need to eat half a cup of cherries in any one day. You may also like to add them to your blender and make a juice.

Baking Soda

Baking soda has been found to be helpful for lowering uric acid levels. When experiencing an acute gout attack, mix half a teaspoon of baking soda in an 8oz glass of water and drink the entire mixture at once. Avoid taking more than 4 teaspoons of baking soda per day, as this may increase the risk of having high blood pressure.

Apple Cider Vinegar

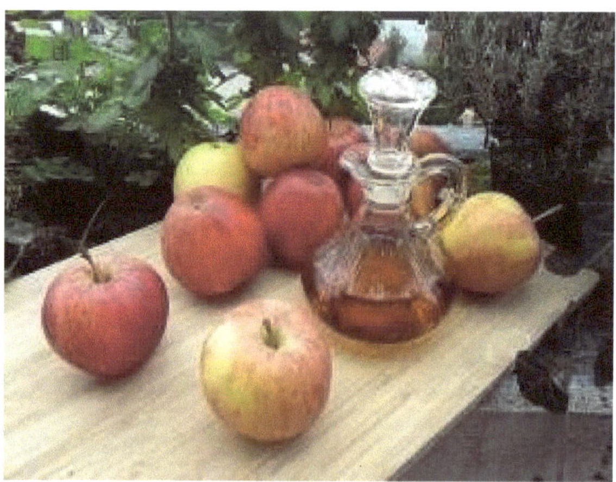

Apple cider vinegar has long been touted to be effective in providing relief from joint pain caused by arthritis and gout.

Apple cider vinegar has an alkalizing effect, therefore providing relief to people suffering from too much acid in the body. It's one of the reasons it's also helpful for relieving heartburn.

For relief from gout pain, just mix one or two tablespoons of apple cider vinegar in a glass of water and drink. When buying apple cider vinegar, make sure it is organic and look for the 'mother web' in the bottle. Then you'll know it's good!

Lemon Juice with Baking Soda

People with gout should try to alkalize their body as naturally as possible. Another way to do this is to drink lemon juice mixed with baking soda. This mixture can help you achieve balanced pH levels.

Combine the juice of one lemon in one half teaspoon of baking soda and wait for the mixture to settle down which may take a few minutes. Then pour the mixture into a glass of water before drinking.

All these natural remedies may prove beneficial in alleviating painful gout attacks.

However, these home remedies, or any other treatment, should not be used as a crutch. Making changes to your diet and lifestyle would be better than any 'fix'. Start making positive changes, especially in your eating habits, followed with healthy lifestyle habits and treat the underlying problem first. Let your pain motivate you to improving your health.

Natural Remedies for Heartburn

There are many natural remedies for heartburn, and many not only relieve your symptoms, but they also help prevent heartburn in the first place. Sufferers will find that what works for one person may not work as well for another, but all it takes is a little trial and error on your part to find the ones that work best for you.

Following are some natural, readily procured ingredients that have relieved the discomfort of heartburn for many people.

Aloe Vera Juice

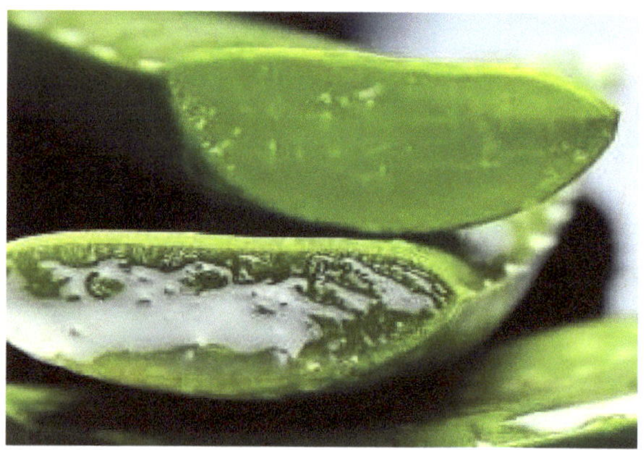

Making a juice out of aloe vera is both soothing to the stomach and is an effective remedy during heartburn attack.

Baking Soda

Baking soda is a known antacid. Studies have shown that baking soda helps to neutralize stomach acid. Drink 1 teaspoon of baking soda dissolved in 8 ounces of water to immediately alleviate heartburn symptoms and acid reflux.

Bananas

Bananas are famous for being a natural antacid. Eat 1-2 fresh or dried bananas to restore healthy acid levels in the stomach.

Chamomile Tea

Stress appears to be strongly correlated to heartburn attacks. To help relieve stress, drink a cup of chamomile tea. The tea also helps to neutralize the acid content of your stomach.

Slippery Elm

Slippery Elm contains substances that can thicken the mucous lining of the stomach thereby creating a barrier against the stomach acid. Pour a few tablespoons of slippery elm extract into a glass of water.

Drink this after having your meals and before going to bed at night.

Ginger or Ginger Tea

One of the oldest natural remedies for heartburn is ginger. It also helps relieve nausea during an attack. Studies have shown that ginger helps regulate the production of stomach acids and gases while you digest, which reduces the amount of acid getting into your esophagus.

Include ginger in your daily diet to prevent further heartburn attacks. Eating some ginger with your meal is enough to do the trick, but if you dislike the taste of ginger you can drink it as tea.

Turmeric

Turmeric is a famous herb used in most curry recipes. Although it might be known as an Asian flavor, it also prevents acid build-up as well as stimulates digestion.

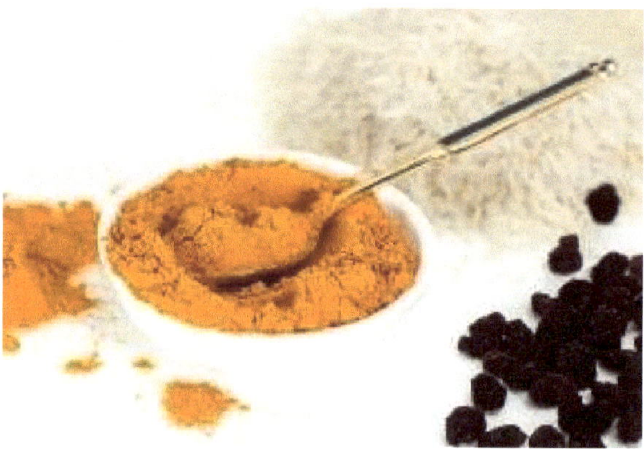

Apple Cider Vinegar

Apple cider vinegar is a popular heartburn remedy. Even though we think of vinegar as being quite acidic, apple cider vinegar has an alkalizing effect on our body. This makes it one of the better remedies that you can choose.

The apple cider vinegar helps neutralize the acids in the stomach, which prevents them from refluxing into the esophagus.

Try a table spoonful in an 8oz glass of water prior to eating, in order to avoid suffering from heartburn. Take the same dose as a remedy to relieve a heartburn attack.

Some people may prefer to take the apple cider vinegar, although this method will definitely make you pucker up! You may have to experiment to find which method works best for you.

Marshmallow Root

Marshmallow contains mucilage which can coat and protect the mucous membrane. When you feel like your throat and chest is on fire, drink a cup of marshmallow solution. Simply mix one teaspoon of powdered marshmallow root into a cup of water and drink your way to relief.

Although over-the-counter medications are convenient, home remedies offer safer preventative measures and they can also save you money. Used properly, natural remedies can stop the pain and discomfort before they even begin.

Natural Remedies for Hemorrhoids

Hemorrhoids are a painful condition often caused by excessive straining during bowel movement, and there are two types - internal and external.

The only difference between an external and an internal hemorrhoid is the location of the hemorrhoid. If it appears in the upper anal canal, it is an internal hemorrhoid, but if it appears in the lower anal canal near the anus and just below the pectinate line, it is termed an external hemorrhoid.

Hemorrhoids are equally prevalent in males as in females. They are also more prevalent in mature people, as the elasticity of the muscular lining in the anal walls deteriorates. The anal wall is more prone to injury due to straining and exertion especially during bowel movement.

Due to the personal nature of this delicate but painful problem, many people search for natural remedies to treat their hemorrhoids. Here are a few which have provided relief to others.

Aloe Vera Gel

An application of aloe vera gel in the anal area once a day will promote healing. It is also soothing and helps with any persistent irritation experienced.

Ice Pack – Not for The Faint-Hearted

Put ice cubes in a cold compress bag and apply this to the affected area. The cold ice provides relief by allowing the veins to shrink. The cold temperature reduces hemorrhoid pain caused by swelling and inflammation.

A word of warning! Don't overdo it by inserting ice cubes into the rectum. You may only worsen your condition and end up with frostbite!

Flax Seeds

Take one tablespoon of ground flax seed up to three times a day. You may also add some flax seeds to your cooking. Eating flax seeds increases your fiber intake, promoting more regular and easier bowel movements.

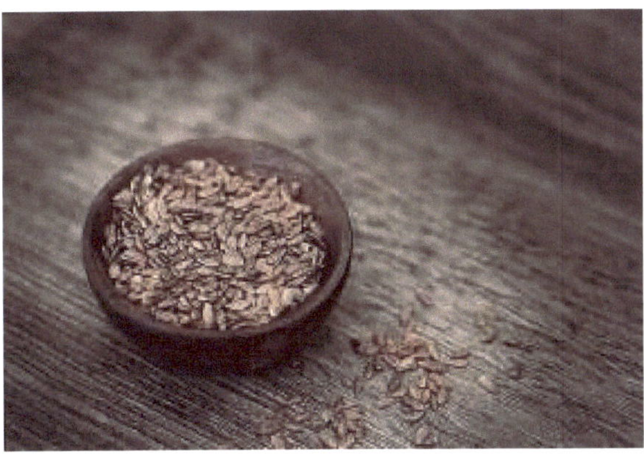

Oak Bark

Cut 50g (1.75 oz.) of Oak Bark into small chunks and place in a liter (quart) of water. Boil for approximately 3 minutes and allow to cool. Pour it into a large basin and sit your backside in the solution for thirty minutes. The warm water will help increase the flow of blood to the rectal area.

The effects become noticeable in as little as a few hours, or can take up to 2 days until relief is found. This method, similar to a sitz bath, will promote circulation of blood in the anal area and will hasten the healing process.

The sitz bath is often recommended and a conventional method of treating hemorrhoids. In a sitz bath, the patient is seated in a bathtub with warm water, enough to cover the anal area. This should be done a couple of times a day for 15 minutes each session.

A warm compress can also be used as an alternative for a sitz bath.

Butcher's Broom

Butcher's Broom extract contains properties that provide relief from inflammation. It also contains ruscogen, a compound that enables the veins to constrict and provide relief for swollen tissues. It can be bought in tea or capsule form.

Avoid Prolonged Sitting

Sitting for long periods of time is claimed to aggravate the condition. If your work requires you to be sitting most of the time, go for a walk whenever you can.

Avoid Lifting Objects That Are Too Heavy For You

Avoid doing tasks that require excessive straining such as lifting heavy objects. Ask someone for assistance, or split the load into manageable portions to avoid excessive straining.

Avoid Salty, Fatty or Sugary Foods

Salty foods such as potato chips, canned foods, and salted nuts may increase your blood pressure and trigger the swelling of your rectal veins.

Foods full of processed sugars may put you at risk of having pressured bowel movements, constipation and rectal or anal irritation.

Foods high in saturated fats may solidify your stools and make bowel movements difficult, therefore further irritating or causing hemorrhoid discomfort.

Alcohol and other indulgences have been linked to hemorrhoids. It is no coincidence that outbreaks are worse following periods of celebration or excess.

A Healthy Diet and Lifestyle for a Healthy Digestive System

Diet changes are recommended for patients with hemorrhoids to avoid dehydration and constipation, that may cause excess straining during bowel movements. Eating plenty of fiber will help regulate bowel movements and prevent constipation, and excessive straining.

Drink plenty of water for proper hydration and softer motions when eliminating, and exercise regularly, as exercise helps the body function properly and contributes to the proper regulation of the bowel.

Hemorrhoids can be prevented through proper diet and exercise. Living healthy and eating healthy is the cure for most 'dis-eases' today. So make your health a top priority!

Natural Remedies for High Blood Pressure

High blood pressure is a growing health issue. While genetics can predispose a person to hypertension, diet and lifestyle are major contributing factors. One widely recognized influence is stress.

There are so many time pressures placed upon us today - no pun intended. Life sometimes feels like a ticking time-bomb and as a result, blood pressure levels can be affected and remain elevated.

Chronic stress and poor diet are often linked and both contribute to high blood pressure. Both are also symptoms and causes of each other – stress increasingly leads to less than ideal food and beverage choices, and eating an excess of simple carb, processed foods increases stress symptoms.

Natural treatment options exist, both for lowering blood pressure and for helping relieve the stress that may be causing it.

Arjuna

Arjuna bark is a good source of CoQ10 (Co-enzyme Q-10), which is another component of many blood pressure and cholesterol supplements. This bark has been used for many years as an important part of Ayurvedic treatment for patients with elevated blood pressure.

CoQ10 plays a crucial role in the proper functioning of the vital organs in the body, especially the heart and liver. The body's own CoQ10 can become depleted as we age. This can result in weaker heart muscles, putting us at risk of developing heart palpitations and high blood pressure. The good news is that these health problems can be prevented by taking natural supplementation of CoQ10, or arjuna bark. The heart will be able to function better and high blood pressure will become less of a problem.

Garlic

One Daily Express headline said, "A daily dose of garlic can save your life." The article related to lowering high blood pressure, not the latest vampire movie.

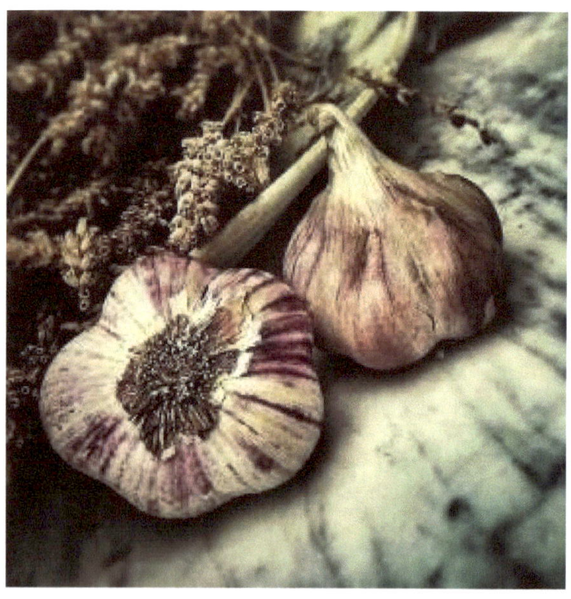

Garlic extract lowers blood pressure because it can stimulate nitric oxide in the cells. This causes the dilation of blood vessels, thereby lowering blood pressure. You will find garlic extract as an ingredient in many natural supplements for high blood pressure because it is such an effective remedy.

Rauwolfia – Indian Snakeroot

Rauwolfia, also known as Indian snakeroot, is a rich source of alkaloids. This herb helps lower blood pressure because its alkaloids help control nerve impulses passing through various nerve pathways. This positively affects the blood vessels and heart, resulting in lower blood pressure.

Apple Cider Vinegar

Apple cider vinegar has been referred to as a miracle cure for lowering high blood pressure, and for its ability to provide fast-acting relief. Taking one tablespoon of apple cider vinegar three times a day, for a week, can help lower blood pressure. If you find it too strong to drink straight, you can have it mixed in a glass of water.

The DASH Diet

This is a diet you may not have heard of. It helps lower high blood pressure.

This diet plan covers the importance of reducing sodium intake, because too much sodium can dramatically increase your blood pressure. A DASH diet has been recommended for people who are sensitive to the adverse effects of salt.

Natural Remedies for Irritable Bowel Syndrome (IBS)

A diagnosis of Irritable Bowel Syndrome means that you have a chronic disorder of the large intestine. Symptoms of IBS might be abdominal pain, gas, constipation, diarrhea, bloating and cramping – all of which can seriously disrupt your lifestyle.

These symptoms can also occur as a result of many other conditions, ranging from mild to dangerous. A specific diagnosis of IBS allows a patient to more specifically avoid the causes and choose effective remedies. It can also be very reassuring to know that the symptoms are not signs of a far more serious ailment.

Although troubling and inconvenient, IBS doesn't increase your chances of colorectal cancer or damage your bowel tissue like Crohn's disease and other colon issues. Also, you can learn to manage and reduce the symptoms by making changes to your diet and reducing stress in your life.

There isn't a single known cause for IBS, but there are several factors which may put you more at risk. A healthy intestine has muscles which move in a relaxed rhythm when food moves from the stomach through the intestinal tract and out of the rectum.

When a person has irritable bowel syndrome, the rhythm is uncoordinated and the contractions of the intestine may be more pronounced causing diarrhea, gas and bloating. The opposite may also occur and the process of moving food through the intestine may be slow and lead to hard and sometimes painful stools.

Try These Natural Remedies

If you have been diagnosed with IBS, you may want to try the following natural methods to reduce the symptoms:

Probiotics – You'll find probiotics (live bacteria) in fermented foods such as yogurt and kefir or in supplements. Some trials indicate that probiotics may help lessen IBS symptoms such as abdominal pain.

Fiber – Fiber found in such foods as fruits, vegetable and whole grains are full of nutrients and vitamins and may make a difference in reducing the symptoms of irritable bowel syndrome.

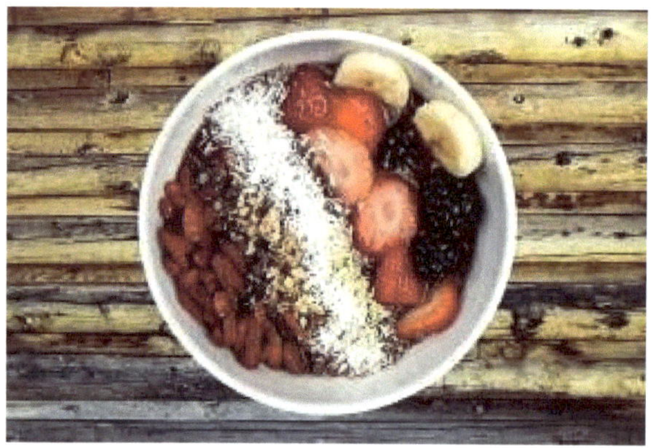

Prebiotics – There are conflicting results for the non-digestible carbohydrates known as prebiotics. Their job is to make sure the good bacteria in your digestive system is fed. Onions, garlic, raw asparagus and bananas can help the microflora in your intestines stay healthy.

Peppermint Oil – Pain resulting from IBS seems to be alleviated by this herbal remedy. It is an anti-spasmodic that can be especially effective in lessening the pain associated with irritable bowel syndrome.

Digestive Enzymes – Supplements of digestive enzymes may be helpful, especially if your main symptom is diarrhea.

The above dietary inclusions can help reduce the intensity of symptoms, and over time reduce the frequency of incidences of IBS. There are also dietary exclusions and lifestyle changes that will prove effective in reducing and even preventing IBS experiences. Instead of tolerating or only treating the symptoms, try the following to free yourself from IBS altogether.

- Lower the stress level in your life.

- Exercise.

- Eliminate foods such as carbonated drinks, raw fruits and some vegetables such as cabbage and cauliflower.

- Adopt a gluten-free diet. This dietary change may help eliminate diarrhea symptoms.

- Eliminate fermentable oligo-di-, monosaccharides and polyols (FODMAPs) from your diet that are present in various grains, dairy and vegetables.

- Carbohydrates such as lactose, fructose and fructans may also contain FODMAPs.

- Get enough sleep.

Compared to prescription medications for IBS, herbal remedies have fewer side effects and are safer for long-term use. If the symptoms of IBS persist after seriously implementing diet and lifestyle changes, seek another diagnosis, to make sure you don't have a more serious condition.

Natural Remedies for Treating Gum Disease

Gum disease is an inflammation or infection that damages the gums. The three stages of gum disease are gingivitis, periodontitis and advanced periodontitis. Dentists see more than three million gum disease cases every year in the United States alone.

Although gum disease requires a medical diagnosis, there are no imaging or lab tests necessary. Symptoms of gum disease might be red, tender and swollen gums and is often caused by poor oral hygiene. If you don't take steps to halt the condition, you could face tooth loss and other health problems.

There appears to be a genetic link to gum disease and some people are far more susceptible than others. If you are one of the unlucky ones, you will have to be more pro-active in your dental self-care. For example, you may have to floss at least daily to prevent plaque buildup, whereas others around may seem to neglect their basic dental hygiene and not suffer.

If you already have gum disease, you can help prevent it from getting worse with improved dental hygiene and maintenance. You can also check out the following methods for helping prevent gum disease to see which might be best for you:

Turmeric Paste and Garlic

Turmeric is a natural anti-inflammatory herb that is part of the ginger genus, and garlic is a known antibacterial agent.

You can either rub cloves of garlic on the irritated gums or make a turmeric and garlic paste and use as toothpaste. Rinse your mouth for a few minutes after using.

Charcoal

Charcoal helps heal gum disease and also whitens the teeth. You wouldn't think that the blackness of charcoal could do that, but it does!

Neem

A plant widely used in India for its antimicrobial and antifungal qualities to promote dental health. You may also be able to find neem in toothpaste or mouthwash.

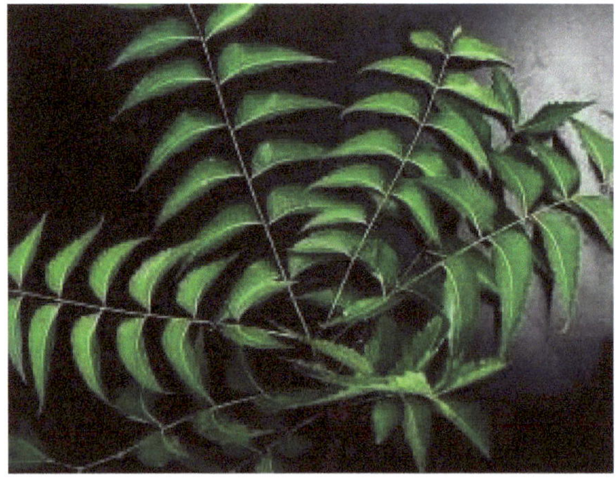

Sage Leaf

Make a decoction out of sage leaves to help avoid gingivitis and gum disease. It's an old folk remedy that is made by boiling about 50 fresh and organic sage leaves in distilled water. Then gargle the liquid several times throughout the day – or you can make a sage tea to drink. The natural antioxidants, anti-inflammatory and antimicrobial properties of sage should provide relief and prevention.

Oil Pulling

Helps to cure red and swollen gums and has even been found to reverse bone loss from gum disease. Oil pulling actually pulls the toxins from your gums by removing plaque buildup. Use 100% organic olive, sesame or coconut oil and swish the oil in your mouth for a few minutes at a time.

Aloe Vera Gel

If you can, use the aloe that comes directly from the plant. It has an anti-inflammatory effect that helps reduce redness and inflammation in gums.

Mustard Oil

This remedy has been used for hundreds of years to destroy bacteria in the mouth that causes gum disease. It not only heals the gums, but helps reduce pain because of its antibacterial and antimicrobial agents.

Eating plenty of fruits and vegetables with skins on them also helps to clean the teeth and prevent gum disease from taking hold. The vitamin C and antioxidants contained in many fruits and vegetables help prevent plaque from building up on the teeth and affecting the gums.

The sooner you address the gum disease issue, the better chance you have of effectively treating the disease without the trauma and danger of more intensive dental procedures.

You may have gum disease developing for a long time without any warning signs, so always take care of your mouth and teeth to ensure good dental health for the rest of your life.

Natural Remedies for Sore Throat

Pharyngitis or commonly known as a sore throat, is an illness we've all experienced. A sore throat is the most common manifestation of a viral infection, but it can also be the result of an infection caused by bacteria.

These can be due to a common cold, influenza, laryngitis, infectious mononucleosis, or mumps. Other infections may be due to a streptococcal infection. It might also be due to tonsillitis or inflammation of the tonsils, epiglottis inflammation, and uvula inflammation.

There are different methods and treatments for sore throats, depending on the causative agent. Since the most common cause of sore throats is due to viral infections, antibiotics are often just a waste of time and money. They don't treat viruses, only bacterial infections. That's why it is important to know what the cause is before taking any medication.

More often than not, we take a sore throat lightly, but it's still nice to alleviate the symptoms with some natural remedies. So, put an end to your suffering by using any of the following natural remedies for a sore throat.

Slippery Elm

The use of slippery elm for treating several conditions such as sore throats and coughs has been adopted by modern herbalists from the Native Americans. Slippery Elm is a tree which is common to North America. It contains mucilage which turns into a slippery gel when mixed with water.

This slippery gel coats a painful sore throat, thereby providing relief. If you are taking any medications, consult your doctor first as slippery elm can also slow down the absorption of some medicines. This is because the slippery substance may coat the digestive system making it difficult for the medications to be absorbed.

Sage Gargle

Use sage solutions for gargling to provide relief for hoarseness and a sore throat. You can purchase sage in a form of liquid extracts, dried leaves or essential oil.

When making sage gargle solutions, pour a cup of hot water on to two teaspoons of sage dried or fresh leaves. After a few minutes, strain, then add a pinch of salt. The extra solution can be kept inside the refrigerator for use later.

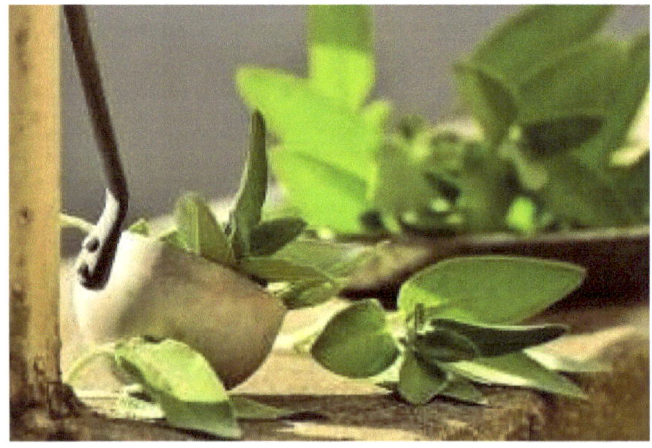

Licorice Root

Licorice root has been used by both Western and Eastern medical traditions for providing relief to people who are suffering from a sore throat, viral infection and ulcers. Licorice contains demulcent properties which are helpful in soothing the mucous membrane of the throat.

It can be purchased in powder, tea, tincture, capsule and extract form. If you want to use its roots, you need to boil in water for a couple of minutes.

Marshmallow Root

This is another demulcent herb that provides soothing and cooling effects to the mucous membranes of the throat.

If you are a diabetic, consult your health care provider before taking any marshmallow root preparation. Marshmallow root contains substances that may lower your blood sugar levels and affect your medications.

Salt Water Solution Gargle

Gargling a warm salt water solution is another classic remedy for a sore throat. Mix half a teaspoon of salt to a glass of warm water. Use this for gargling every four to five hours. This warm solution can also be helpful in breaking down the hard and sticky phlegm caused by a common cold.

Apple Cider Vinegar and Salt Gargle

Another effective gargle is an apple cider vinegar and salt gargle. In a half glass of lukewarm water, add a pinch of salt and a few teaspoons of apple cider vinegar.

Use this mixture a couple of times a day, especially when you wake up and before you go to bed. The salt will act as an antiseptic and the vinegar relieves the pain and soothes inflammation quickly.

Drink Plenty of Cool Water

Avoid drinks that are too hot as they will increase any inflammation. Instead, drink plenty of cool water and suck on ice cubes to diminish an inflamed throat.

Vitamin C and Citrus Fruits

Make sure you are getting plenty of vitamin C, either through citrus fruits or supplements. Vitamin C promotes faster healing and helps fight against infection.

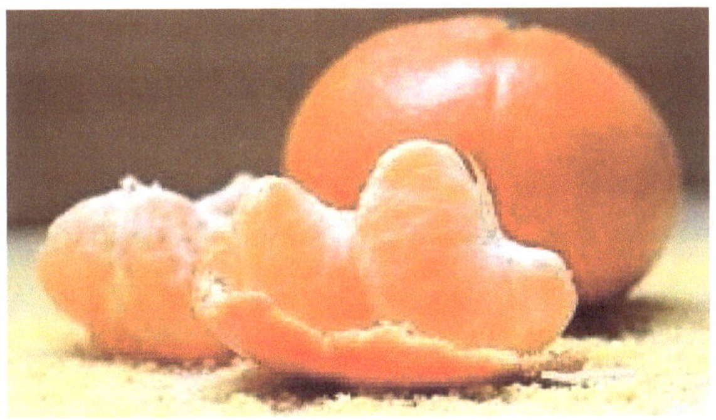

Garlic

Garlic is a powerful antibiotic and antiseptic. It will reduce inflammation, relieve pain, and help fight off infection. Eat raw cloves and add to your meals to get daily health benefits.

Although a sore throat is not a serious or life-threatening disease, it certainly is a nuisance. Keeping these natural remedies handy will at least help you get rid of your sore throat and find relief faster.

Natural Remedies for Tinnitus

Tinnitus is the technical term used to describe the incessant ringing or buzzing sound in the ears. This ringing sound can only be heard by the patient.

Tinnitus is not a disease but a condition, and may be a symptom of an underlying and more dangerous health problem. It can be a one sign of neurological problems like multiple sclerosis. It can also denote an ear infection, fluid build-up due to nasal allergies, or wax build up in the middle ear.

Types of Tinnitus

Pulsatile tinnitus is like hearing sounds like that of a heartbeat, your own pulse, or muscle contractions. Muscular movements near the ear, any changes in the ear, or blood flow problems in the neck or facial area may create these sounds.

Nonpulsatile tinnitus is caused by the cochlear or auditory nerves, the nerves responsible for hearing.

The most common reason a person develops tinnitus is due to hearing loss or from frequent exposure to excessively loud noises or sounds. If work-related, this is known as industrial deafness.

Quite often tinnitus just comes and goes, and doesn't require medical intervention. However, if it gets worse and affects both ears, it would be wise to get it checked to make sure it is not a sign of any underlying problem.

Herbal and Dietary Remedies

When you are confident that it is not, you might like to use the following natural remedies for tinnitus to reduce the annoying ringing in your ears.

Ginkgo Biloba

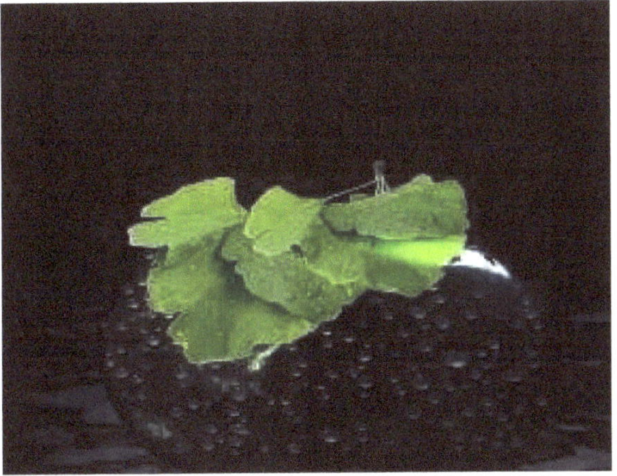

This herb tops the list of natural remedies for tinnitus. Its active compounds have been found to be effective in improving several functions of the circulatory system. It helps improve the blood flow, especially to the peripheral areas of the body, making ginkgo biloba an excellent tonic. It can be an especially good remedy for tinnitus if the main cause of tinnitus is due to circulatory problems.

Avena Sativa

This herb comes from a wild oat plant which can be used effectively as a nervous system tonic. Avena sativa also works well in maintaining healthy cholesterol levels and benefiting the circulatory system.

Rosmarinus officinale

This is another invigorating herb which works well as a nerve tonic. Its active constituents are helpful for promoting the health of the blood vessels, which is important for tinnitus sufferers.

This herb also improves mood and energy levels, helping an individual cope better with stress, which helps lessen the symptoms of tinnitus.

Verbena officinalis

This herb is popular for its ability to relieve the effects of stress and for helping achieve balance and harmony. Its active compounds support the overall health of the nervous system.

Vitamin B12

Vitamin B12 can help treat tinnitus as it is an essential vitamin for nerve ending health and it protects the neurons from inflammation that might cause tinnitus.

Food sources include, fresh pineapples, garlic, and sea vegetables. Otherwise vitamin B12 supplements may be helpful. Vitamin B12 helps reduce inflammation and prevents the hardening or stiffening of the bones in the middle ear, that may cause a ringing or buzzing sound.

Other Treatment Options

Cranio-Sacral Therapy

This is hands-on therapy designed for improving the flow of cerebral spinal fluid within the spinal column and brain. A skilled cranio-sacral therapist can usually help reduce the symptoms of tinnitus in just one session.

Tinnitus Retraining Therapy - TRT

This therapy teaches tinnitus sufferers how to get rid of their negative emotional reactions towards tinnitus. An individual who undergoes Tinnitus Retraining Therapy will be able to learn better coping skills in dealing with their tinnitus.

Do's and Don'ts

Avoid food that triggers tinnitus such as chocolates, dairy products, foods high in cholesterol and fat, and salt, as these can exacerbate tinnitus symptoms.

Eat high protein foods, fresh fruits and vegetables, olive oil, coconut oil, and nuts.

Importantly, avoid or reduce stress at all cost as it can make problems worse.

A major cause of tinnitus is the lack of supply of blood and oxygen to the ears. Taking vitamins and supplements that improve blood circulation and reduce inflammation on the nerve endings may prove extremely helpful.

Eating a healthy diet and regular physical activities will improve blood circulation and regulate supply of blood and oxygen to the ears.

Natural Remedies for Urinary Tract Infections (UTI)

Sometimes referred to as bladder infection, urinary tract infections are a condition characterized by the frequent urge to urinate, and a painful, burning sensation during and after urinating.

If bacteria affects either the kidney or the ureters, it is classed as an upper urinary tract infection. If it affects the bladder or the urethra, it is referred to as a lower urinary tract infection.

Women are more susceptible to developing a UTI due to their physiologic or body structure. The location of the woman's urethra is very near the anus which makes it easier for the bacteria to travel to the urinary tract. Sexual activities can also make them more susceptible. A history of diabetes, pregnancy or insufficient water intake will increase risks of a UTI occurring.

At the onset of symptoms, it's important to take prompt treatment action to avoid further complications such as a kidney infection. You can take remedial action right away with a few natural remedies listed below.

Cranberries

Cranberries top the list of the most popular remedies for urinary tract infections. The cranberry juice contains a natural antimicrobial property – proanthocyanidins - that fight off invading organisms and keeps the body healthy.

It prevents bacteria from reaching the urethra walls. It also has mild antibiotic effects. The antibacterial effects of cranberry juice can be present in the urine for hours after the last intake.

It is recommended to take pure cranberry juice, about half a glass daily. This amount is enough to keep infection at bay. In the absence of pure cranberry juice, cranberry supplements may prove helpful.

Blueberries

Blueberries are another member of the "berry" family that is known to be effective in relieving the symptoms of Urinary Tract Infections. Blueberries contain bacteria inhibiting properties.

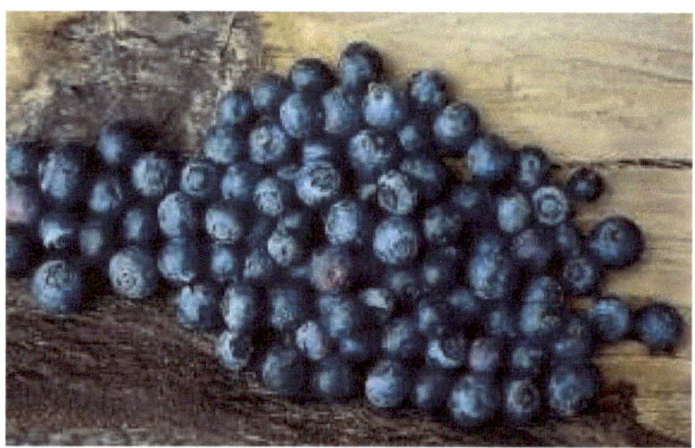

Regular consumption of blueberries helps prevent the growth of bacteria, so drink a glass of blueberry juice in the morning and at night for faster relief from UTI symptoms. You may like to add some fresh blueberries to your morning cereal or mix some blueberries in your cranberry juice.

Goldenseal

Goldenseal is another herb that can nip UTI in the bud. It contains plant alkaloids known as berberine that improves the immune system and eliminates the bacteria that caused the infection.

Uva Ursi

For thousands of years, Uva ursi has been used by Native Americans and the Chinese in treating Urinary Tract Infections. It is an herb that contains arbutin, a substance that is converted to hydroquinone in the urine that provides an antiseptic effect. Uva Ursi is also a diuretic herb that helps in flushing out the bacteria from the kidneys.

If you are under Uva Ursi treatment, make sure you replace your potassium levels, as you may become deficient as you flush away fluids from your body.

Apple Cider Vinegar

Apple cider vinegar contains potassium and other enzymes that are helpful for treating UTI and preventing the bacteria from multiplying. Apple cider vinegar also contains active compounds that act as antibiotics.

Add two or three teaspoons of apple cider vinegar to a glass of water every day to prevent urinary tract infections and promote good health!

Baking Soda

Baking soda helps to neutralize the acidity of the urine. Add a teaspoon of baking soda to a glass of water. This will help relieve the symptoms of UTI and lead to faster recovery.

Drink Plenty of Water

The importance of adequate hydration, even more than normal, cannot be overstated. Quite often a person with a UTI tries not to drink as it is painful to urinate. Don't do this!

Water helps flush the bacteria out. Make sure you drink at least 8 glasses of water every day. Apply a hot water compress on your lower abdomen to ease the burning sensation when urinating.

Pineapples

Pineapples are a rich source of bromelain that helps reduce inflammation caused by a urinary tract infection. It also contains vitamin C that boosts your body's ability to fight off the infection. Regularly eating a cupful of pineapple can help prevent the recurrence of a UTI.

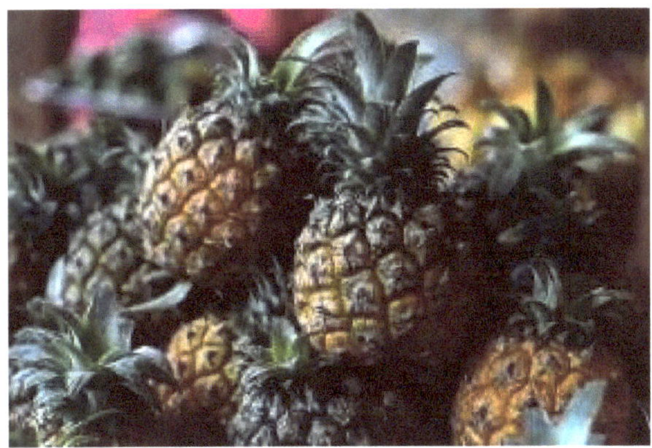

Eat fresh pineapple juice instead of canned products that may contain preservatives, or take bromelain supplements if fresh pineapples are out of season.

Vitamin C

Vitamin C is an excellent vitamin for boosting the immune system and protecting against many infections. For people who have recurrent urinary tract infections, doctors may recommend taking at least 5,000 mg of vitamin C daily.

Vitamin C can easily be obtained from food sources, such as citrus fruits, papaya, guava, watermelon, kiwi fruit and raspberries, however when large dosages are required supplementation may be necessary. Consuming these types of foods will create an environment that is not conducive for bacteria and pathogens to grow.

Diuretic Herbs

There are plenty of herbs that can be used as part of your urinary tract infection treatment plan. One example is the horsetail plant which has diuretic properties, which hastens the recovery of a UTI through an increased urine flow. As more urine passes through the bladder, more the bacteria are flushed away.

Other examples of plants that have diuretic properties include hydrangea and dandelion. Parsley is also an herb that can promote urination and at the same time reduce inflammation.

Urinary tract infections can be greatly avoided by eating a healthy diet rich with food sources the bacteria can't live in, drinking plenty of water, and watching hygiene practices.

Final Thoughts

Most of the treatments can be very effective in reducing the intensity of symptoms. Some can help reduce the incidence of the condition occurring, and even help prevent it altogether.

Not all treatments are medicinal, but as you have read, some are as much about what you should not eat. Some others are non-dietary but are actions and steps you can take for yourself to reduce the impact of your particular health problem.

We have been conditioned by the pharmaceutical industry, with its almost unlimited advertising budget, to think that we need a prescription drug or over the counter medication to fix our various ailments.

Hopefully this document has helped you realize that natural home remedy options do exist, are readily available, and in many cases work as well or better than the commercial alternative, but without a lot of undesirable side effects.

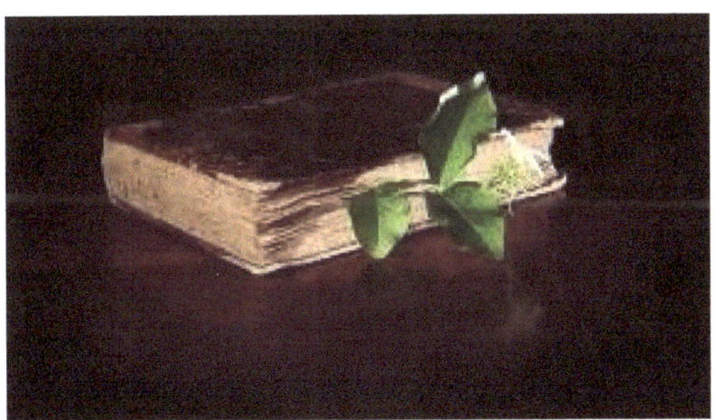

Other Relevant Books by This Author

If you would like to read more relevant books about this topic, here is a list of the CreateSpace links, titles and descriptions from this author:

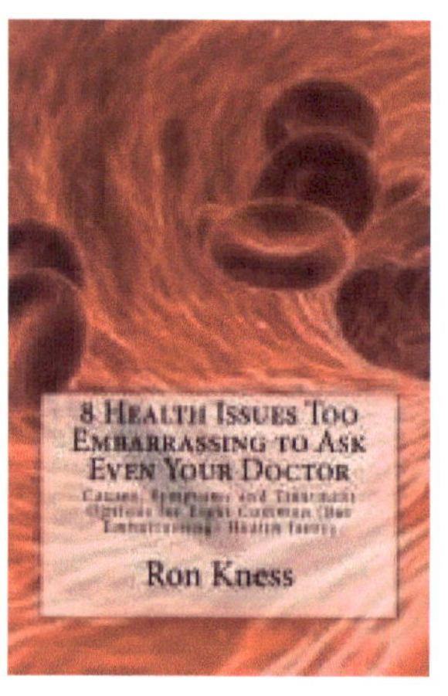

https://www.amazon.com/Health-Issues-Embarrassing-Even-Doctor/dp/1544827490

8 Health Issues Too Embarrassing to Ask Even Your Doctor: Causes, Symptoms and Treatment Options for Eight Common (But Embarrassing) Health Issues

In this book, we look at all of the ways you can improve your own health through the identification and treatment of these embarrassing health issues, starting with reading about what causes the condition, its symptoms and treatment options not involving prescription medications or doctor intervention.

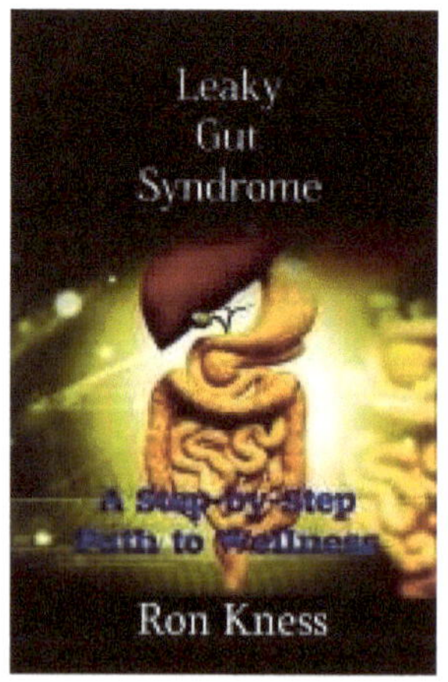

https://www.amazon.com/Leaky-Gut-Syndrome-Step--Step/dp/1537314823

<u>Leaky Gut Syndrome - Could This Be Why You Are Sick?: A Step-by-Step Path to Wellness</u>

Leaky gut is just now starting to come onto the radar for doctors as more and more people are developing gastrointestinal and other disorders with no known cause.

If you have frequent unexplained sickness, you could have leaky gut syndrome. What it means is things are getting through the wall of the small intestine that aren't supposed to get through.

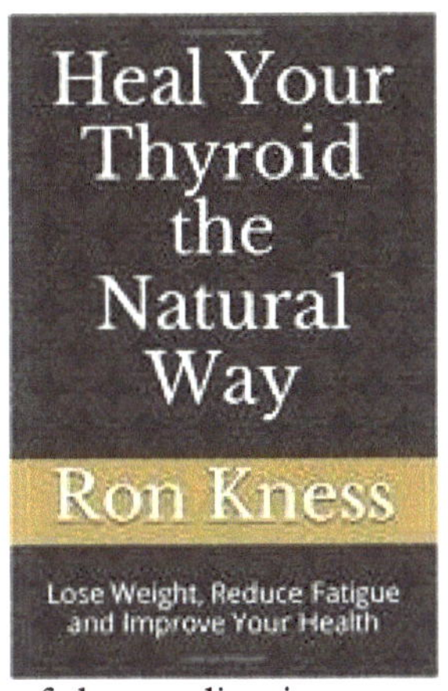

https://www.amazon.com/Heal-Your-Thyroid-Natural-Way/dp/1520544030

Heal Your Thyroid the Natural Way: Lose Weight, Reduce Fatigue and Improve Your Health

Having great thyroid health through proper nutrition and exercise is linked to not wanting to rely on taking a lot of medications. This is because the side effects of the medications can be worse than the conditions they treat. In this book, we look at all of the ways you can improve your own thyroid health through nutrition and exercise, starting with getting tested to see if your thyroid is working properly or not in the first place.

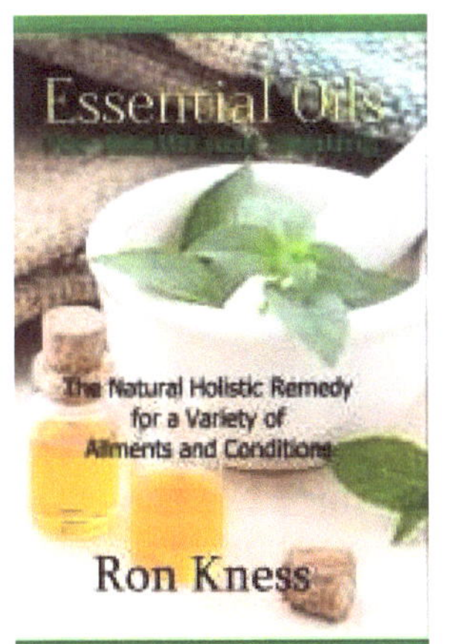

https://www.amazon.com/Essential-Oils-Health-Healing-Conditions/dp/1542359007

<u>Essential Oils for Health and Healing: The Natural Holistic Remedy for a Variety of Ailments and Conditions</u>

Essential oils can not only help you with some health issues, but they could end up being your natural holistic remedy for headaches and migraines, joint aches and pains, chronic pain, menstrual irregularities, cuts, scrapes and burns, signs of aging and wrinkles, anxiety and depression If you have never used essential oils before, get a starter kit and start using them.

About the Author

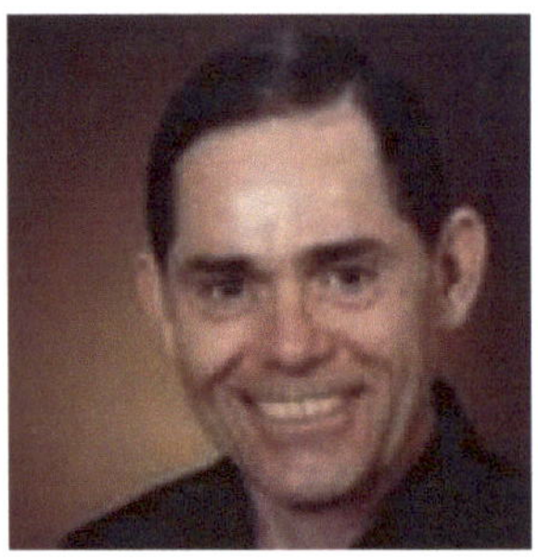

I have published over 125 books on Amazon for Kindle, CreateSpace and other publishing platforms.

While most of my books are on health and fitness in general, as I age (now 65) at the time of this writing) my topics of interest are geared toward aging baby boomers and older.

Besides my own writing, I also ghostwrite ebooks, books, reports, articles, blogs and do Kindle conversions for clients on a variety of topics.

Today my wife and I are retired from our careers and live in Gold Canyon, AZ. I now write as a retirement business where you'll find me happily sitting in my office typing away on my laptop as I work on my next book or ghostwriting project . . . that is if we are not traveling on a cruise ship - our new-found mode of travel.